S.O.S Oily - Combination Skin

Marta Pueyo Sastre

S.O.S Oily - Combination Skin

Marta Pueyo Sastre

S. O. S
Oily - Combination Skin

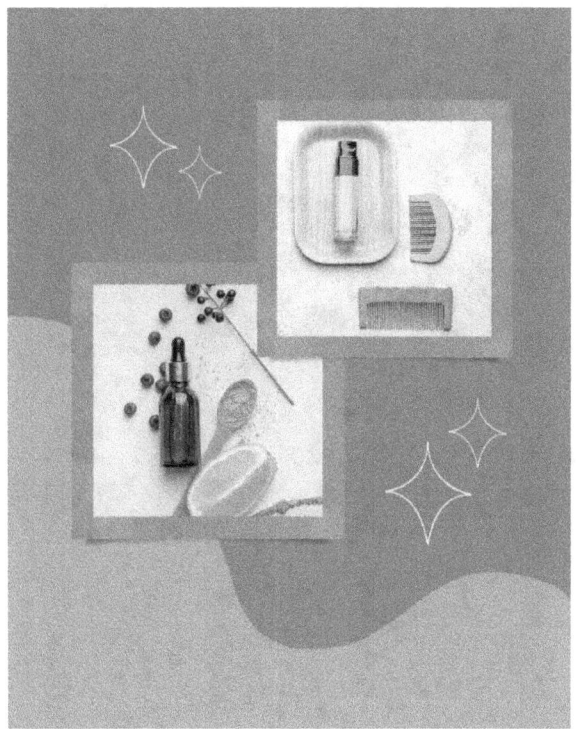

Marta Pueyo Sastre

INTRODUCTION

If you have oily or combination skin, you've come to the right place. Here, you will find all the advice you need to manage excess sebum and other associated issues, such as acne and inflammation. We will also discuss various other related topics.

You, like me, know that having this type of skin can be a hassle—sometimes even a torment. However, I want to encourage you and share all the knowledge I've acquired over the years on this subject, as well as help you through my experience to achieve greater well-being.

There are many types of skin, but for everyone, it constitutes the largest organ of the body. Therefore, we must take proper care of it to keep it healthy and provide us with good protection.

In this concise manual, a brief anatomical overview of the skin is presented, along with its functions and the layers that comprise it. I believe it is important to understand, even if not in great depth, how our precious skin works.

We will also differentiate between what we mean when we talk about combination skin and oily skin, because although they are similar concepts, they have their differences and thus require slightly different and specific care.

There are various skin conditions, and here we will focus on acne—its formation process, the risk factors that increase this problem, and the difference between common acne and acne vulgaris, among many other things.

The market offers a wide variety of specific products to solve this problem. We will discuss the most effective ones, both chemical and natural. While these topical substances help significantly in treatment, we must also take care of ourselves from the inside. The healthier we are, both physically and psychologically, the better our external physical appearance will be.

I hope this guide helps you and that you can consult it whenever you need.

Sincerely, Marta, your healthcare professional.

INDEX

1. The skin__pg.7

2. What is oily skin and combination skin?__pg.14

3. How and why does acne occurs?__pg.16

4. Types of acne__pg.17

5. Polycystic ovary syndrome__pg.19

6. Scars and spots__pg.20

7. Products and active ingredients__pg.23

8. Natural remedies__pg.26

9. Skincare routine__pg.29

10. Conclusions__pg.31

THE SKIN

Our entire body is covered with skin and, as we said at the beginning, it is the largest organ we have (it measures 2 m2 and weighs approximately 5 kg). It also has various functions.

Its thickness varies depending on the body area, for example, on the eyelids it measures 0.5 mm, and on the heels, 4 mm.

It constitutes the separation between the external and internal environment and therefore protects us against external aggressions, as well as microorganisms, which have a harder time entering our body.

For this reason, we must avoid as much as possible carrying open wounds. In this way, it contributes to maintaining all the structures of the body intact while acting as a communication system with the environment.

The baby's skin is thinner than that of an adult, and in adolescence, it becomes oilier due to the activity of the sebaceous glands caused by hormonal changes, and as a consequence, acne may appear.

At the age of 40, it becomes drier and less elastic, and wrinkles appear; and in older people, many wrinkles and spots appear.

Men's skin produces more sebum than women's because they produce more androgens, which are the male sex hormone, so their skin is thicker and oilier.

The cutaneous adnexa, which are the nails, hairs, and sebaceous and sweat glands, depend on it.

The skin can also suffer from different diseases, such as dermatitis, seborrhea, and acne.

There are different types of skin depending on the body area where it is located:

→**Thin or soft:** It is on the eyelids and genitals. He has no lucid stratum.

→**Thick:** Lip, soles, palms. With highly developed, lucid, grainy, spiny, and basal strata.

The skin is mostly made up of the following cells:

√ **Keratinocytes**: They are segmented in the stratum corneum.

√ **Melanocytes or pigmentoncytes:** They give pigmentation to the skin and they are on the germ layer.

Under histological sections of the skin, the following can be seen:

- Langerhans cells
- Lymphocytes
- Mechanoreceptors or Merkel cells

We can highlight the following functions of the skin:

- **PROTECTION:** Covers and protects tissues and serves as a defensive barrier against pathogens. It also prevents water loss.

- **THERMAL REGULATION:** Allows the body to adapt to changes in temperature, both external and internal.

Regulation is done through blood vessels, sweat glands, adipose tissue, and the structure of the skin.

The sweat glands are located in the dermis and communicate with the exterior through pores through which sweat escapes.

Together with sweat, heat, and waste substances are eliminated.

- **DRYING AND EXCRETION**: Sweat comes out through the sweat glands, and sebum is produced through the sebaceous glands.

- **ABSORPTION**: The skin is impermeable to water and permeable to lipids (ointments...).

- **RECEPTION**: Receives signals from the outside (touch, pain, temperature, pressure) and transmits them to the brain.

- **SYNTHESIS**: Vitamin D is formed from ultraviolet light hitting the skin.

- **IS INVOLVED IN THE IMMUNE RESPONSE.**

We also need to know what parts of the skin are divided into:

✓ **EPIDERMIS**: This is the most superficial layer of the skin; it has no blood vessels or nerves. It is thicker on the soles of the feet and palms of the hands. It is, in turn, made up of several layers, which, from the innermost to the most superficial, are:

- **Basal or germinative stratum**: This is the innermost layer. This is where the new cells that will replace those of the upper stratum are formed. It is also made up of melanocytes, which are the cells that give the body its tan.

- **Stratum spinosum.**

- **Stratum granulosum.**

- **Lucidocyte:** It has a very thin zone with eosinophilic features, which is involved in the immune response. The nuclei begin to degenerate in the outer cells of the granulosa and disappear in the luteal cells.

- **Stratum corneum:** The outermost and thickest stratum corneum is made up of dead cells overlaid with keratin.

As the lower strata grow, new cells are generated and push the older, upper cells upwards until they slough off and fall away; this is how the cells are renewed, and this process occurs every four weeks.

✓ **DERMIS:** This is the middle layer of the skin, which is thicker and is made up of connective tissue.

It contains blood vessels, lymphatics, nerve endings, sweat and sebaceous glands, and hair follicles.

Like the epidermis, it is divided into layers:

*PAPILLAR DERMIS: It has protrusions or papillae, which correspond to those of the epidermis; these are the fingerprints.

*RETICULAR DERMIS: It is deeper and contains collagen that gives the skin strength and elasticity.

- Nerve endings can be:

    - **Nociceptors**: pain receptors.

    - **Thermoreceptors:** Temperature receptors.

    - **Mechano-receptors**: touch receptors.

- It also contains corpuscles, which collect sensations:

    - **De Paccini**: They pick up vibrations and pressure.

    - **Ruffini's**: They pick up the sensation of heat.

    - **De Meissner:** They pick up the sensation of fine touch. They are on the palms of the hands, soles of the feet, fingertips, lips, tip of the tongue, nipples, glans, and clitoris.

    - **De Krause**: They pick up the sensation of cold.

    - **Merkel's**: They pick up the sensation of superficial touch.

✓ **HYPODERMIS**: This is the deepest layer of the skin. It is made up of adipose tissue, i.e., fat-producing cells called lipocytes. It is criss-crossed by collagen, blood vessels, and nerves.

Sebum is beneficial for the skin as it lubricates the skin and prevents it from drying out, but an excessive increase is detrimental and will result in skin problems.

Collagen is the most abundant component in the skin; it gives smoothness and is a protein substance, i.e., it is a protein.

SKIN APPENDAGES

They are structures that develop from the dermis, receive nutrients, electrolytes, and fluids from the dermis, and are released through the epidermis.

❖ **NAIL:** These are epidermal productions in the shape of a sheet, formed by keratin. They cover the back of the distal phalanges, protecting the toes.

They are made up of:

- **Cuticle**
- **Lunula**
- **Nail body**

❖ **HAIR:** These are keratin stalks that form in a hair follicle and consist of:

- **Stem:** Visible part
- **Root:** internal part. It is inside the hair follicle, at the end of which there is a dilatation called the bulb.

❖ **GLANDS**

- **Apocrine sweat ducts:** In axillae, genital area, areolas, and nasal vestibule.

Their duct ends in a hair follicle. Thicker and more odorous secretion.

- **Eccrine sweat:** They are found almost everywhere on the body. They predominate on the palms, soles, feet, and armpits. Their duct ends on the outside through the pores.

- **Sebaceous:** Produce sebum and end up in the infundibulum of the hair follicle. There is no hair where there is hair. Sebum keeps the skin supple and waterproof.

PATHOLOGIES ASSOCIATED WITH THE SKIN

As mentioned above, there are many pathologies associated with the skin. About acne, it is important to be aware of some of them and to know how to differentiate acne lesions from other infectious processes, which will require other types of treatment.

o **PURPLE:** This is an alteration in the colouring of the skin, in the form of reddish patches of vascular origin.

o **PAPULA:** *A solid lesion less than 1 cm in diameter (acne).*
o **NODULE:** A solid lesion with an elevation of 1 to 2 cm, affecting the dermis and epidermis. They are painful, hard, and very inflamed and reach deep layers of the skin.
o **RONCH:** A solid lesion, with elevation and oedema around it. Itchy. Mosquito bites or allergic processes.
o **VESICULA:** A lesion with an elevation of less than 1 cm in diameter with fluid.
o **AMPOLLA:** A lesion larger than the gallbladder, with fluid more than 1 cm in diameter.
o **PUSSULA:** A lesion with fluid (pus), with a well-defined elevation. Blister with pus.
o **COSTRA OR POSTILE:** Desiccation of blood, serum, or pus on the surface.
o **CYCATRIX:** New tissue formation whose purpose is to repair a loss of substance. We will discuss them in more detail below and look at the different types.
o **FOLICULITIS:** Bacterial infection of hair follicles caused by Staphylococcus, usually affecting shaved areas.
o **FORUNCULO:** Staphylococcal bacterial infection of 1 or more hair follicles. In areas with abundant hair, and where there is a lot of friction and sweat (buttocks, armpits, nape of the neck).

- **HYPERKERATOSIS:** Overproduction of keratin and dead cells. It can also clog the pore, so a mechanical exfoliation once a week is advisable.
- **BLACK SPOTS:** Open blackheads. Their blackish colour is due to the oxidation of the lipid material when it comes into contact with the environment.
- **WHITE SPOTS:** These are closed comedones that do not contain pus, and, as their contents do not oxidise as they are not in contact with the exterior, they are white.

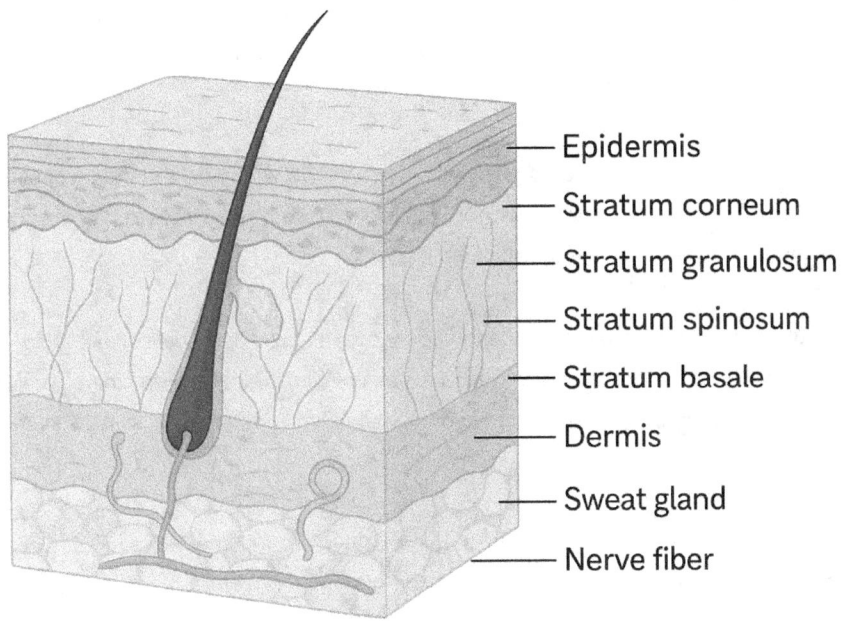

WHAT IS OILY SKIN AND COMBINATION SKIN?

We all want to have healthy, acne-free skin, so we often resort to facial treatments that don't work or even make the problem worse.

Most of the time, this happens because we opt for products that are not suitable for our skin type.

For this reason, it is essential to know what type of skin we have, and in this case, to know whether we have combination or oily skin, so that we will be more accurate when buying, for example, a moisturising cream.

The type of skin we have is determined above all by our genetics, but also by environmental factors in our daily lives, such as the climate in the area where we live, our usual diet, the amount of water we drink, habits such as smoking or alcohol, and many other things.

If we find it difficult to know for sure what type of skin we have, seeing a dermatologist can help.

- **MIXED SKIN**
Combination skin is a combination of dry areas on the cheeks and oilier areas, especially on the forehead, chin, and nose, which we call the T-zone.
Normally, this skin type is determined by genetics, but it is common when using facial products with irritating ingredients that turn normal skin into combination skin by stimulating the sebaceous glands.
It is prone to dry patches and rosacea, but others may also have blemishes and acne, as in oily skin.

- **FAT SKIN**
Oily skin is characterised by thick, oily skin, enlarged pores, and a constant shine.
It is prone to mild to severe acne on the face, neck, chest, back, and shoulders, as well as being easily inflamed and reddened.
It is common among adolescents due to changes in their endocrine system, but it can last a lifetime.

One way to differentiate between the two skin types is by measuring the amount of oil secreted in certain areas of the face.

The face should be washed and left in the open air without any cream for about an hour, and at the end of this time, the entire T-zone should be wiped with toilet paper, for example.

If the paper absorbs oil from that area, but does not pick up oil from other areas, the person has combination skin. In the case of combination skin, the paper will absorb oil from all parts of the face.

Another method is to examine pore size and skin quality. The person with combination skin will observe a smooth facial texture, medium-sized pores, and a healthy colour, while the person with oily skin will observe a shinier facial surface, larger pores, as well as blemishes, blackheads, and acne.

Both skin types need different care, although the moisturiser in both cases should be oil-free.

HOW AND WHY DOES ACNE OCCUR?

Acne is an inflammatory disease of the pilosebaceous unit, i.e., the sebaceous gland leading to the hair follicle, affecting the seborrhoeic areas of the face and trunk.
A blockage of the follicular orifice is caused by excessive retention of sebum, keratin, etc., which is then colonised by Propionibacterium bacteria, causing the pores to become inflamed.
It is most common from puberty to young adulthood, but can last a lifetime.
At this time of life, there is an increase in androgens, which are the male sex hormones; then sebum secretion increases, and the size of the pore increases and becomes blocked. Later the duct is colonised by the bacterium Propionibacterium acnes, which grows and reproduces inside the blocked pore, increasing inflammation and infection, leading to acne.

Factors favouring acne include:
- Hormones: Androgens, corticoids...
- Medications: Contraceptives, lithium, antidepressants, anti-epileptics....
- Toxics: Oils, tars...
- Greasy cosmetics.
- Stress.

It is a highly variable and polymorphic pathology, with several types of lesions coexisting in the same patient:

- Comedones: open and closed, as an initial lesion (inflammatory lesion).
- Follicular papules and pustules in the inflammatory form.
- Inflammatory nodules and cysts: related to a greater depth of follicular inflammation.
- Atrophic or hypertrophic scars.

TYPES OF ACNE

Acne is a very common problem in society.

There are several types of acne, including the following:
- **Acne Conglobata:** Nodulocystic form.
- **Acne Fulminans**: It is accompanied by general symptoms such as fever, arthralgias, bone alterations...
- **Acne vulgaris:** Comedones or papulopustules predominate.
- **Other:** corticosteroid, cosmetic, excoriated...

Acne can be divided into three groups:
1. **Infantile, juvenile, cystic, conglobate, and menopausal acne.**
2. **Exogenous acne:** Caused by drugs, cosmetics, Acne Venenata (due to industrial products).
3. **Endocrine acne:** The acne that occurs in Cushing's disease and polycystic ovary syndrome.

Grades:
- **Grade 1. Mild acne:** The main lesions are blackheads and non-inflamed blackheads. Sometimes there may also be some inflammation, but no more than 5 inflammatory lesions on each half of the face.
There are usually no after-effects.
- **Grade 2. Moderate acne**: In addition to pimples and blackheads, there are between 6 and 20 inflammatory lesions on each half of the face.
- **Grade 3. Severe acne**: Between 21 and 50 inflammatory lesions are found on each half of the face and are also common on the torso and back.
In this case, there will be permanent scarring due to the deep lesions and inflammatory effect.
- **Grade 4. Very severe acne:** More than 50 inflammatory lesions are found on both sides of the face, in addition to papules and pustules, nodules, and cysts.

Types:

- **VULGAR ACNE**

It is the most common and can be divided into different stages depending on the severity of the injuries caused.
It is caused by genetic inheritance, infections, and natural hormonal problems.

- **IATROGENIC ACNE**

It is caused by certain drugs such as steroids, anabolic steroids, testosterone, and androgens.
These drugs cause hormonal imbalances, especially an overproduction of androgens, which stimulate the sebaceous glands.

- **KELOID ACNE OR SCLEROSING FOLLICULITIS OF THE NAPE OF THE NECK**

It is due to poor healing after an inflammatory event, leading to the formation of fibrous plaques, papules, and alopecia.
It is similar to cystic acne and is caused by genetics.

- **ACNE NEONATORUM**

It occurs in newborns in the facial area, where comedogenic and pustular lesions appear.
It is due to hormonal stimulation of the immature pilosebaceous glands.
This is something we would point to as normal, but they are more likely to experience severe acne vulgaris at other stages of their lives.

- **ROSACEA**

Its cause is unknown, but it is known that its formation has nothing to do with regular acne, and it is thought that severe sunburn, stress, anxiety, certain foods, and environmental factors can cause it.

POLYCYSTIC OVARY SYNDROME

This syndrome affects women of childbearing age and is characterised by an overproduction of androgens.

The menstruation of these women is very irregular due to ovarian dysfunction, which can lead to infertility.

It is aggravated by an increase in insulin resistance, with a consequent risk of developing diabetes mellitus.

In addition to this, cutaneous manifestations are very unsightly, such as acne, hirsutism, alopecia...

Regarding acne, we can say that it occurs in almost half of the cases of this syndrome.

We can be suspicious when the acne is late, i.e., in people over 25 years of age or in severe or persistent acne.

Androgens increase sebum secretion by the sebaceous glands and cause alterations in follicular keratinisation, which promotes acne.

Many studies have shown a relationship between acne severity and androgen levels in the blood, although in certain cases the level of androgens is normal, whereby androgens are produced and secreted locally in the sebaceous gland due to a hypersensitivity of the follicle to androgens or an overactivity of the androgen-producing enzymes in the sebaceous gland.

If you have the symptoms mentioned above, it is advisable to see a doctor to rule out this pathology.

SCARS AND SPOTS

The healing of acne depends on the previously existing lesions, which vary in their depth and inflammatory process.

Deep pimples have a complicated healing process and leave permanent scars on the skin, which can be of different types.

The face is the most visible part of our body, so it often affects the biopsychosocial sphere, i.e., it affects both the physical, psychological, and social spheres.

Once they appear, it is very difficult to eliminate them, so it is logical to think that the best prevention is to prevent the appearance of acne.

The dermis, which, as we have seen at the beginning, is the middle layer of the skin, is mostly made up of collagen and elastin, which are proteins that give volume, elasticity, and texture to the skin. It is also the layer that contains the sebaceous glands, so the infectious process greatly affects this layer.

During the repair process of an acne lesion, new dermal tissue has to be formed, which has been destroyed during the inflammatory process of the pimple.

> ✓ **Macules (marks)**: This type is the mildest, as it involves a change in the colour of the skin, rather than its texture. They are similar to spots that are darker or lighter than our skin colour, and although they take time to disappear (months), they can be achieved by chemical, mechanical, and enzymatic exfoliation with different products.
> They can be purplish, white, brown, or reddish and can be prevented by daily use of sunscreen with a sun protection factor of 50 or higher.
> Superficial chemical peeling treatments can be performed in the beauty clinic, as well as at home with products such as salicylic acid, glycolic acid, pyruvic acid, or tretinoin.
> What this exfoliation does is to accelerate the replacement of the epidermal surface layer cells, so that they gradually fade and disappear.
> Another option that dermatologists can use is LED light, always after assessment of the patient.

✓ **Hypertrophic or keloid scars:** These types of skin lesions are formed when an excessive amount of collagen is produced during the healing process.

In hypertrophic wounds, the new tissue does not extend beyond the wound margins, but in keloids it does.

They are the most difficult to treat and occur after intense inflammatory (nodulocystic) acne, and can also cause pain, itching, and tightness, although they are more frequent in areas of the body other than the face, such as the back and trunk.

Some therapeutic options are local corticosteroid infiltration, laser light, or, in very severe cases, surgical intervention as a last resort.

✓ **Atrophic scars:** These scars are characterised by a kind of hollowing or hollowing of the skin because the new collagen fibres have been arranged incorrectly, producing shallower depressions at the sites of previous inflammatory acne lesions.

Depending on their shape, they are classified into different types:

- o *Wavy or Rolling*: They are shaped like dunes.
- o *Van or boxcar*: They have a depth of more than 1 mm in diameter.
- o *Ice pick*: Beak-shaped, but less than 1 m in diameter.

There are different treatments to treat the different types of sequelae, but they all aim to increase collagen synthesis to fill in the gaps.

For example, deep peels, dermabrasions, laser systems, hyaluronic acid fillers, and dermapen.

<u>Treatments for acne scars can be differentiated into two types:</u>

- **Ablative treatments**: These consist of removing the superficial layers of the skin, destroying them chemically or physically to promote a new healing process from the deep layers of the skin and regenerate the affected areas.

They can cause burns and pain, and it is essential to use sunscreen during treatment, which can last from weeks to months, as well as painkillers and antibiotics.

  - Deep peelings.
  - Dermabrasions: A skin rejuvenation procedure that uses a rotating device with burs to remove the epidermis, which is the outermost layer

of the skin. The new skin will then be smoother, and scars and blemishes will fade.

- CO_2 laser systems.

• **Non-ablative treatments:** This type of treatment helps regenerate collagen without causing injury to the skin, such as fractional lasers.

Each type of treatment will be decided by the doctor or dermatologist, depending on the type, extent, and location of the lesions.

PRODUCTS AND ACTIVE INGREDIENTS

The care routine should be adapted to the severity and type of injury.

Proper hygiene should be carried out every day, morning and evening. If we are consistent, the results will be noticeable.

We can distinguish:

- ❖ **Topical products**: Home routine is key to controlling excessive sebum secretion and the appearance of acne.

    - ☐ **Benzoyl peroxide**: This can be found in cream or gel format. It has an antimicrobial, comedolytic, and antibacterial action, which makes it very effective against the bacteria involved in the process of acne formation.

    - ☐ **Retinoic acid (retinol/isotretinoin)**: Retinoids are forms of Vitamin A. They are small molecules that penetrate the dermis and promote cell renewal, fade blemishes, and stimulate the formation of collagen and elastin.
    It is very effective for oily skin, as it has a sebum-regulating action, and it mattifies the skin, reducing shine and unclogging pores.
    They should be used at night.

    - ☐ **Cleansing soaps**: They must regulate excessive oil secretion and prevent blackheads, so they will include in their formulation some active ingredients that help to achieve this, such as salicylic acid, among others.
    To be used daily, morning and evening.

    - ☐ **Mechanical exfoliators**: These contain hard particles that remove dead cells and promote cell renewal. They should be used approximately twice a week. They should be indicated for oily or combination skin, so that they also have a comedolytic effect.

    - ☐ **Enzyme peels**: This is one of the gentlest exfoliating treatments. It uses plant enzymes to break the bonds between dead cells and remove them without damaging the living cells. This reduces blemishes, refines fine lines...

☐ **Chemical exfoliants**:

Alpha hydroxides (AHAs) are water-soluble and come from natural products.

Beta hydroxides (BHA) are fat-soluble and therefore penetrate the skin through the pilosebaceous follicles, which is why they are most suitable for oily skin and acne.

Finally, polyhydroxyacids (PHA) are also water-soluble, but have larger particles, so their action is more superficial.

> o **Salicylic acid (BHA)**: Regulates sebum formation, reduces skin inflammation, and improves acne. It has an antiseptic and exfoliating action.
>
> o **Glycolic acid (AHA):** It comes from sugar cane or beetroot. It renews cells, refines pores, lightens blemishes, and fills wrinkles.
> For people with sensitive skin, daily use should be limited to avoid redness and flaking.
>
> o **Azelaic acid (AHA):** It comes from cereals such as wheat, barley, or rye and is one of the most effective. It treats hyperpigmentation, acne, and inflammation, and has antibacterial action.

☐ **Vitamin C:** A powerful antioxidant, it also has an antibacterial and anti-inflammatory effect. It provides luminosity and reduces hyperpigmentation. Protects against free radicals.

In addition, it helps produce collagen, so it also plays a role in mitigating the effects of ageing.

☐ **Moisturising creams:** We cannot forget to moisturise our skin, as many people mistakenly believe that because they have oily skin, they should not do so.

They should be oil-free and non-comedogenic to avoid clogging pores, but still provide good moisturisation.

There are many more products on the market; here are the ones that have worked best for me, after a long time testing different active ingredients.
You should find the ones that suit you best and adapt your routine to your case.

❖ **Oral:** This refers to drugs such as antibiotics, hormones, etc. It must always be taken under medical prescription.

NATURAL REMEDIES

Natural and home remedies are a good alternative and a good complement to the products mentioned in the previous section.

They are cheaper and less aggressive for the skin, but we should still consult a specialist.

One of these alternatives is the use of medicinal plants, specifically the following, which have been studied and are effective:

- **ALOE VERA**

This plant is frequently used in the cosmetics industry. In particular, the pulp obtained from its leaves is added to various products such as soaps and creams.

It has many benefits for various skin conditions, including acne.

It can be applied directly to the skin and left to act for a few minutes or together with other ingredients such as honey, in the form of a mask.

These benefits and properties include:
- Antiseptic and antibacterial properties.
- Contributes to wound healing.
- It has an anti-inflammatory effect, so it repairs tissues.
- Moisturises.
- Calming effect.
- Prevents ageing.
- Astringent property, eliminates excess grease.

- **BARDANA**

This herb has an anti-inflammatory effect and is taken as an infusion.

- **SQUID**

It is a yellow flower widely used to treat skin conditions such as eczema or acne, thanks to its soothing and repairing properties, as well as its anti-inflammatory and antiseptic properties. We can also find soaps that contain it, which provide extra hydration.

- **ECHINACEA:** It belongs to the daisy family. It can be taken in infusions, or essential oils can be applied to the skin.

- **BREWER'S YEAST**

It can be consumed or applied topically as a mask together with other ingredients.

- **TEA TREE**

It is one of the most effective essential oils for combating acne, as it has antiseptic, antifungal, and anti-inflammatory properties.

- **NIAULI**

It is another very useful essential oil for this condition.

- **MUSK ROSE**

In this case, it is used to treat the marks and fade them, but not to treat the cause of the acne.

Other natural products include:

- **HONEY**

Honey has several benefits, such as antiseptic and antibacterial properties, which is why professionals consider it a good alternative for treating skin problems.

We can apply it to the skin in the form of a mask, even together with other ingredients with active properties against this type of problem.

- **LEMON**

It also has antimicrobial effects and is an antioxidant. It lightens the skin, so it is also useful for treating marks.

Phytotherapy is the use of medicinal plants for the natural treatment of different ailments in the human organism. In this case, to treat mild or moderate acne, using plants such as those seen above, which have antibacterial, astringent, depurative, and other effects.

Among the most useful plants are aloe vera, pansy, and burdock, and they generally have fewer significant adverse effects than pharmacological treatments, as well as providing our bodies with various vitamins and benefits.

We should be aware that most of the cosmetic products we use daily contain ingredients that are very harmful to our health.

There is currently a lot of concern about this issue, and therefore, applications have been created that tell us whether the ingredients of a product are really suitable for health or, on the contrary, toxic.

These products, when used over a long period of time, cause systemic effects. They can be neurotoxic, endocrine disruptors, and even carcinogenic.

Some of them are:

- **Sodium Lauryl / Laureth Sulfate (SLS and SLES):** It can be found in toiletries such as facial soap, among others. It is absorbed through the skin and accumulates in organs such as the heart, brain, eyes, and liver, causing long-term problems such as cataracts or corrosion of hair follicles, among many other harmful effects.

- **Parabens (isobutylparaben, butylparaben, methylparaben, propylparaben):** These are found in almost all personal care products. They can alter hormone levels, as happens with oestrogen, which causes an alteration in the endocrine system, which is very important in the development of breast cancer. They can also cause rosacea, infertility...

- **BHA and BHT:** Can be found in moisturisers, as well as in a multitude of products. They are antioxidants that extend the life of products, but they are carcinogenic, endocrine disruptors, and cause liver damage.

- **EDTA (ethylenediaminetetraacetic acid):** Toxic to organs and tissues.

These four substances are just one example of a huge list of such products, which can make us sick in the long run. More and more brands are launching natural products that do not contain ingredients that are harmful to our health. They are usually more expensive, but it is worth it. Other brands can mislead us; they can sell a product as natural when, in fact, if you read the ingredients label, it is the opposite.

SKINCARE ROUTINE

A proper skin care routine and thorough cleansing are key to maintaining the highest level of skin health.

In this case, we must choose the right products for oily or combination skin so that they are effective against this problem and we do not aggravate it unnecessarily.

1. **Cleansing:** This is the first and most important step, especially for this type of skin. It ensures that the skin is free of impurities, environmental pollution, and excess oil and thus avoids clogged pores, because if this happens, acne will appear.
Milk formats should be avoided as they contain some oil, and non-comedogenic products should be used.
Double cleansing consists of first wiping with a cotton pad soaked in micellar water specifically for this type of skin and then washing with water and a cleanser in gel or tablet form. This cleansing is recommended for this type of skin as it cleanses in depth.

2. **Mechanical exfoliation:** Chemical or enzymatic exfoliation is more advisable in the case of sensitive skin. But in this case, it should be done once or twice a week to avoid over-drying the skin.
An exfoliating scrub should also be used that is suitable for this skin type.

3. **Toner**: Specially for our skin, to help tighten pores and balance the pH.

4. **Serum**: Such as vitamin C.

5. **Moisturising cream**: This is very important as it reinforces the skin's protective barrier and maintains moisture, which is essential.
For oily skin, oil-free, non-comedogenic gel formats should be used, as well as antiseptic ingredients.

For combination skin, light creamy textures are always non-comedogenic and sebum-regulating.

5. **Sunscreen factor 50:** Always apply sunscreen half an hour before leaving the house in the morning after moisturising cream and repeat every 2 hours, so that the skin is protected to the maximum and thus avoid spots and acne marks. As it is not advisable to use make-up on oily and combination skin, there are protective creams with colouring, so at the same time, they protect us from the sun's rays, we conceal blemishes and marks.

6. **Masks:** Once or twice a week, it is recommended that after exfoliation, we apply a mask. We can make one at home with natural products or a commercial one, for example, with green clay.

7. **Chemical exfoliants**: They are recommended to be used at night in the routine before going to bed, before the moisturiser. Glycolic acid in gel format is a very good option, both every night and every two or three days, for more sensitive skin.

In addition to topical care, we should exercise for at least half an hour a day, and shower as soon as possible to clean the pores and prevent them from clogging.

Likewise, we should eat a balanced diet, avoiding processed foods, sugars, carbohydrates, etc.

CONCLUSIONS

As we have seen, we have a multitude of treatments that will help us have more beautiful skin.

If you are one of those people who think that because you have oily skin, it is impossible to do anything about the signs of ageing, you are wrong, this type of skin needs specific care, but it is not because you have an excessive production of sebum that you have to leave aside moisturising, counteracting blemishes, scars and wrinkles.

Many of the products I have detailed have anti-acne, anti-wrinkle, and anti-spot functions, and we can benefit from all the advantages they offer.

Each of us must know the type of skin we have and the most appropriate hygiene and care routine for that type of skin, as well as limiting the factors that increase production and being consistent in doing so throughout our lives, as the predominance of the disease is not only in adolescents, but can extend to different stages of life.

The following aspects should be borne in mind:
o It is absolutely contraindicated to squeeze or scratch the lesions, as this will worsen the problem and cause wounds that will also become infected.
- o Avoid using cosmetics with a high fat content. They should always be non-comedogenic or oil-free.
- o Consult your doctor if you are taking medication, as this could worsen the problem.
- o Eat a varied diet, avoiding fats, alcohol, and tobacco.
- o Shave smoothly.
- o Cleaning makeup brushes
- o During exfoliation treatment, skin peeling occurs. Always do it gently.
- o Always follow the treatment prescribed by our doctor. Never self-medicate.
- o Bear in mind that it is a long treatment, that you must be patient, always following the indications.
- o Medicines for this problem are usually expensive, as are cleansers and moisturisers.

o It involves changing our habits and acquiring new ones.

Throughout the reading we have seen that there are different types of acne and different classifications of this problem. All of them cause aesthetic problems and in many people who have this pathology or who have to live with its after-effects, they can present psychological problems and social isolation.

While mild acne can be treated with skin care alone, more severe forms require oral medications such as antibiotics to kill the infection present in the epidermis internally.

These pharmacological treatments are very aggressive for our organism, so they can only be taken under medical prescription, when the professional, given the patient's characteristics, considers it appropriate and necessary.

There are infectious skin conditions that can be confused with acne, so if you have any doubts, the best option is to see a dermatologist, so that he or she can establish a true diagnosis and an appropriate treatment.

Remember, healthy skin is radiant skin. Take care of it as soon as possible, and don't forget the sunscreen even on cloudy days.

Here are some activities I propose to you.

I challenge you to write:

- Your daily hygiene habits and routine.
- If you know your skin type.
- If you knew how acne occurs and what types there are.
- How often do you go to the dermatologist.
- The cosmetic products that work for you and the ones you have tried.
- General skin condition.
- Characteristics of your skin.
- Alcohol and tobacco use.
- Usual type of diet.
- What would you like to improve or what habits would you like to acquire?

Then I ask you to think about whether there really is something you are doing wrong or are simply not doing to improve and maintain your skin in an optimal state.

Good luck!

I wish you all the best in this complicated yet beautiful journey called life.

© **El Arte De Cuidar. All rights reserved.** No part of this content may be reproduced, in whole or in part, by any means without the prior written consent of the author.

www.ingramcontent.com/pod-product-compliance
Lightning Source LLC
Chambersburg PA
CBHW071842210526
45479CB00001B/255